RENAL DIET
BREAKFAST AND SNACKS
COOKBOOK

*Improve your kidney health
with low potassium and
low sodium recipes.
Quick and easy recipes
for beginners*

Charlotte Smith

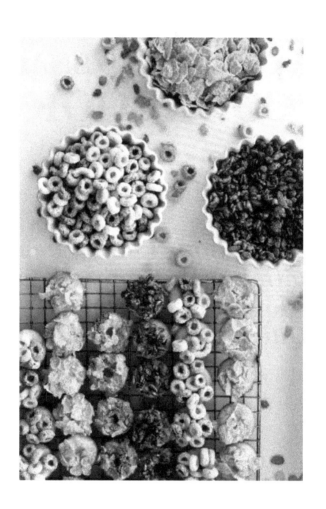

Table of Contents

Additionally, the information in the following pages is intended only for informational purposes and should thus be thought of as universal. As befitting its nature, it is presented without assurance regarding its prolonged validity or interim quality. Trademarks that are mentioned are done without written consent and can in no way be considered an endorsement from the trademark holder.

Introduction

Kidney disease is becoming more prevalent in the United States, and so we need to learn as much about it as we can. The more we educate ourselves, the more we can do to take care of this important bodily system. If you've been diagnosed with chronic kidney disease (CKD), education can empower you to most effectively and purposefully manage the disease. Once you have a full knowledge of what chronic kidney disease is, you can begin to take charge of your evolving health needs. Making healthy changes early in the stages of kidney disease will help determine how well you will manage your kidney health. I am here to guide you, every step of the way. Like any new process, it may seem intimidating at first.

What Do the Kidneys Do?

Our kidneys are small, but they do powerful things to keep our body in balance. They are bean-shaped, about the size of a fist, and are located in the middle of the back, on the left and right sides of the spine, just below the rib cage. When everything is working properly, the kidneys do many important jobs such as:

- Filter waste materials from the blood
- Remove extra fluid, or water, from the body
- Release hormones that help manage blood pressure
- Stimulate bone marrow to make red blood cells
- Make an active form of vitamin D that promotes strong, healthy bones

What Causes Kidney Disease?

There are many causes of kidney disease, including physical injury or disorders that can damage the kidneys, but the two leading causes of kidney disease are diabetes and high blood pressure. These underlying conditions also put people at risk for developing cardiovascular disease. Early treatment may not only slow down the progression of the disease, but also reduce your risk of developing heart disease or stroke.

Kidney disease can affect anyone, at any age. African Americans, Hispanics, and American Indians are at increased risk for kidney failure, because these groups have a greater prevalence of diabetes and high blood pressure.

When we digest Protein, our bodies create waste products. As blood flows through the capillaries, the waste products are filtered through the urine. Substances such as Protein and red blood cells are too big to pass through the capillaries and so stay in the blood. All the extra work takes a toll on the kidneys. When kidney disease is detected in the early stages, several treatments may prevent the worsening of the disease. If kidney disease is detected in the later stages, high amounts of Protein in your urine, called macro albuminuria, can lead to end-stage renal disease.

The second leading cause of kidney disease is high blood pressure, also known as hypertension. One in three Americans is at risk for kidney disease because of hypertension. Although there is no cure for hypertension, certain medications, a low-sodium diet, and physical activity can lower blood pressure.

The kidneys help manage blood pressure, but when blood pressure is high, the heart has to work overtime at pumping blood. When the force of blood flow is high, blood vessels start to stretch so the blood can flow more easily. The stretching and scarring weakens the blood vessels throughout the entire body, including the kidneys. And when the kidneys' blood vessels are injured, they may not remove the waste and extra fluid from the body, creating a dangerous cycle, because the extra fluid in the blood vessels can increase blood pressure even more.

With diabetes, excess blood sugar remains in the bloodstream. The high blood sugar levels can damage the blood vessels in the kidneys and elsewhere in the body. And since high blood pressure is a complication from diabetes, the extra pressure can weaken the walls of the blood vessels, which can lead to a heart attack or stroke.

Other conditions, such as drug abuse and certain autoimmune diseases, can also cause injury to the kidneys. In fact, every drug we put into our body has to pass through the kidneys for filtration.

An autoimmune disease is one in which the immune system, designed to protect the body from illness, sees the body as an invader and attacks its own systems, including the kidneys. Some forms of lupus, for example, attack the kidneys. Another autoimmune disease that can lead to kidney failure is Good pasture syndrome, a group of conditions that affect the kidneys and the lungs. The damage to the kidneys from autoimmune diseases can lead to chronic kidney disease and kidney failure.

Treatment Plans for Chronic Kidney Disease (CKD)

The best way to manage CKD is to be an active participant in your treatment program, regardless of your stage of renal disease. Proper treatment involves a combination of working with a healthcare team, adhering to a renal diet, and making healthy lifestyle decisions. These can all have a profoundly positive effect on your kidney disease—especially watching how you eat.

Working with your healthcare team. When you have kidney disease, working in partnership with your healthcare team can be extremely important in your treatment program as well as being personally empowering. Regularly meeting with your physician or healthcare team can arm you with resources and information that help you make informed decisions regarding your treatment needs, and provide you with a much needed opportunity to vent, share information, get advice, and receive support in effectively managing this illness.

Adhering to a renal diet. The heart of this book is the renal diet. Sticking to this diet can make a huge difference in your health and vitality. Like any change, following the diet may not be easy at first. Important changes to your diet, particularly early on, can possibly prevent the need for dialysis. These changes include limiting salt, eating a low-Protein diet, reducing Fat intake, and getting enough calories if you need to lose weight. Be honest with yourself first and foremost—learn what you need, and consider your personal goals and obstacles. Start by making small changes. It is okay to have some slip-ups—we all do. With guidance and support, these small changes will become habits of your promising new lifestyle. In no time, you will begin taking control of your diet and health.

Making healthy lifestyle decisions. Lifestyle choices play a crucial part in our health, especially when it comes to helping regulate kidney disease. Lifestyle choices such as allotting time for physical activity, getting enough sleep, managing weight, reducing stress, and limiting smoking and alcohol will help you take control of your overall health, making it easier to manage your kidney disease. Follow this simple formula: Keep toxins out of your body as much as you can, and build up your immune system with a good balance of exercise, relaxation, and sleep.

Stages of Kidney Disease

Based on the United States National Kidney Foundation, kidney disease can be classified into five different progressive stages. These stages and their symptoms do not only help the doctor to devise an appropriate therapy but also guide the patient to take the necessary measures in routine life. The rate of kidney function actually tells much about these phases. In the early stages, there is minimum loss of function, and this loss increases with every stage.

The eGFR is used as a standard criterion to measure the Kidney function. EGFR is the acronym for the estimated Glomerular Filtration Rate. It is the rate at which the waste material is transferred from the blood to the nephron's tubes through "glomerulus"- the filtering membrane of the kidney tissues. The lesser the rate of glomerular filtration, the greater the problem the kidneys are going through. A person's age, gender, race, and serum creatinine are entered into a mathematical formula to calculate his eGFR. The serum creatinine level is measured in a blood test. The creatinine is actually a waste product of the body which is produced out of muscular activities. Healthy kidneys are capable of removing all the creatinine out of the blood. A rising creatinine level is therefore a sign of kidney disease. It is said that if a person has been having an eGFR of less than 60 for three months, it means that he is suffering from serious renal problems.

There are five major stages of chronic kidney disease, and it can be categorized as follows:

Stage 1:

The first stage starts when the eGFR gets slightly higher than the normal value. In this stage, the eGFR can be equal or greater than 90mL/min

Stage 2:

The next stage arises when the eGFR starts to decline and ranges between 60 to 89 mL/min. It is best to control the progression of the disease at this point.

Stage 3:

From this point on, the kidney disease becomes concerning for the patient as the eGFR drops to 30-59 mL/min. At this stage, consultation is essential for the health of the patient.

Stage 4:

The stage 4 is also known as Severe Chronic Kidney Diseases as the eGFR level drops to 15-29 mL/min.

Stage 5:

The final and most critical phase of chronic renal disease is stage 5, where the estimated glomerular filtration rate gets as low as below 15 mL/min.

Role of Potassium, Sodium, and Phosphorus

1. Sodium

Sodium is considered the most important electrolyte of the body next to chloride and potassium. The electrolytes are actually the substance that controls the flow of fluids into the cells and out of them. Sodium is mainly responsible for regulating blood volume and pressure. It is also involved in controlling muscle contraction and nerve functions. The acid-base balance in the blood and other body fluids is also regulated by sodium. Though sodium is important for the health and regulation of important body mechanisms, excessive sodium intake, especially when a person suffers from some stages of chronic kidney disease, can be dangerous. Excess sodium disrupts the critical fluid balance in the body and inside the kidneys. It then leads to high blood pressure, which in turn negatively affects the kidneys. Salt is one of the major sources of sodium in our diet, and it is strictly forbidden on the renal diet. High sodium intake can also lead to Edema, which is swelling of the face, hands, and legs. Furthermore, high blood pressure can stress the heart and cause the weakening of its muscles. The build-up of fluid in the lungs also leads to shortness of breath.

2. Potassium

Potassium is another mineral that is closely linked to renal health. Potassium is another important electrolyte, so it maintains the fluid balance in the body and its pH levels as well. This electrolyte also plays a vital role in controlling nerve impulses and muscular activity. It works in conjugation with the sodium to carry out all these functions. The normal potassium level in the blood must range between 3.5 and 5.5mEq/L. It is the kidneys that help maintain this balance, but without their proper function, the potassium starts to build up in the blood. Hyperkalemia is a condition characterized by high potassium levels. It usually occurs in people with chronic kidney disease. The prominent symptoms of high potassium are numbness, slow pulse rate, weakness, and nausea. Potassium is present in green vegetables and some fruits, and these ingredients should be avoided on a renal diet.

3. Phosphorus

The amount of phosphorus in the blood is largely linked to the functioning of the kidneys. Phosphorus, in combination with vitamin D, calcium, and parathyroid hormone, can regulate the renal function. The balance of phosphorous and calcium is maintained by the kidneys, and this balance keeps the bones and teeth healthy. Phosphorus, along with vitamin D, ensures the absorption of calcium into the bones and teeth, where this mineral is important for the body. On the other hand, it gets dangerous when the kidneys fail to control the amount of phosphorus in the blood. This may lead to heart and bone-related problems. Mainly there is a high risk of weakening of the bones followed by the hardening of the tissues due to the deposition of phosphorous and calcium outside the bones. This abnormal calcification can occur in the lungs, skin, joints, and arteries, which can become in time very painful. It may also result in bone pain and itching.

What is Renal Diet?

A renal diet is an eating plan exercised to help minimize waste products' levels in the blood. The renal diet is designed to cause as little work or stress on the kidneys as possible, while still providing energy and the high nutrients the body needs.

A renal diet follows several fundamental guidelines. The first is that it must be a balanced, healthy, and sustainable diet, rich in natural grains, vitamins, fibers, carbohydrates, omega 3 fats, and fluids. Proteins should be adequate, but not excessive.

Accumulates in the blood are kept to a minimum. Blood electrolyte levels are monitored regularly, and the diet corrected. It is essential to follow specific advice from your doctor and dietitian.

Daily Protein intake is essential to rebuild tissues but needs to be kept to a minimum. Superfluous proteins need to be broken down by the body into nitrates and carbs. Nitrates are not employed by the body and have to be excreted via the kidneys.

Carbs are an important source of energy and should be taken in adequate amounts. Whole grains are the best. Avoid highly refined carbohydrates.

Table salt ought to be limited to cooking only. Excess salt overworks the kidneys and causes fluid retention. Salty foods like processed meats, lots of foods, sausages, and snacks should be avoided.

Phosphorus is essential for the body to function, but dialysis can't remove it, so amounts need to be monitored, and intake should be restricted though not eliminated completely.

Foods, like dairy products, darker drinks such as colas and legumes, have high phosphorus content. If levels of this increase in the blood, foods high in potassium such as citrus fruits and dark, leafy green lettuce, carrots or apricots might have to be restricted.

Omega 3 fats are a significant part of any healthy diet. Fish is an excellent source. Omega fats are important for the body. Avoid trans-fats or hydrolyzed fats.

Fluids should be enough but might need to be limited in cases of fluid retention.

A healthy renal diet can help keep kidney function for longer. The main differences between a renal diet and any nutritious diet plan are the limitations placed on Protein and table salt ingestion. Restrictions on fluids and potassium might become necessary as signs and symptoms of accumulation become evident.

For people with diabetes who also suffer from kidney disease, there is a food strategy or diet. Over fifty percent of chronic kidney disease sufferers are people that have diabetes, indicating the necessity for them to stick to the diabetic diet.

In several cases, this diet is prepared and is effective in different phases of this disease. There are also instances where the diet is created for people with diabetes hoping to avoid renal disorder. Sufferers of diabetes and kidney problems have trouble eating the proper food.

The aim of a diabetic's meal plan would be to get the blood within the safe selection. This may be carried out just by having meals frequently on a daily basis, not missing any, and eating carbohydrate foods that are low glycemic.

Consuming a number of such carbohydrates at every meal can assist the body in maintaining a moderate blood sugar level, becoming neither too high nor too low.

Low glycemic foods include brown rice, sweet potatoes, and whole-grain bread. But if it is a renal diet for diabetics, whole-grain bread and sweet potatoes ought not to be used since they're rich in potassium.

For people with kidney issues, they should eat less of these foods full of potassium, phosphorus and sodium. A blood sugar-lowering diet for people with diabetes can be a diet suitable for renal issues. Patients need to check labels since sodium is common in several foods.

For clients with kidney problems, dietitians advice against the consumption of diet pops of java because such drinks contain sodium.

On a diabetic-renal meal plan, unsweetened teas, water and diet sodas are allowed. When it comes to vegetables, broccoli, cauliflower, beets, eggplant, and cabbage are usually recommended because of their abundant vitamin content and very low carbohydrate and potassium content. Meats that are rich in sodium, such as organ meats, sausage, and bacon, ought not to be taken.

Since canned vegetables contain lots of sodium, it is necessary to choose raw vegetables and steer clear of the canned variety. Furthermore, raw vegetables are more nutritious, considering their vitamins.

It is recommended that people with diabetes learn from certified nutritionists the foods that they need to eat or avoid.

However, all forms of renal diet have one thing in common, which is to improve your renal functions, bring some relief to your kidneys, as well as prevent kidneys disease at patients with numerous risk factors, altogether improving your overall health and wellbeing. The grocery list we have provided should help you get ahold of which groceries you should introduce to your diet and which groups of food should be avoided in order to improve your kidneys' performance, so you can start from shopping for your new lifestyle.

You don't need to shop many different types of groceries all at once as it is always better to use fresh produce, although frozen food also makes a good alternative when fresh fruit and vegetables are not available.

As far as the renal diet we are recommending in our guide, this form of kidney-friendly dietary regimen offer solution in form of low-sodium and low-potassium meals and groceries, which is why we are also offering simple and easy renal diet recipes in our guide. By following a dietary plan compiled for all stages of renal system failure unless the doctor recommends a different treatment by allowing or expelling some of the groceries, we have listed in our ultimate grocery list for renal patients.

Before we get to cooking and changing your lifestyle from the very core with the idea of improving your health, we want you to get familiar with renal diet basics and find out exactly what his diet is based on while you already know what is the very core solution found in renal diet – helping you improve your kidney's health by lowering sodium and potassium intake.

The best way of getting familiar with renal diet and basics of this dietary regimen is to take a look at the most commonly asked questions that extend the answer to a question what is renal diet?

Benefits of Renal Diet

If you have been diagnosed with kidney dysfunction, a proper diet is necessary for controlling the amount of toxic waste in the bloodstream. When toxic waste piles up in the system along with increased fluid, chronic inflammation occurs and we have a much higher chance of developing cardiovascular, bone, metabolic or other health issues.

Since your kidneys can't fully get rid of waste on their own, which comes from food and drinks, probably the only natural way to help our system is through this diet.

A renal diet is especially useful during the first stages of kidney dysfunction and leads to the following benefits:

Prevents excess fluid and waste build-up

Prevents the progression of renal dysfunction stages

Decreases the likelihood of developing other chronic health problems e.g. heart disorders

Has a mild antioxidant function in the body, which keeps inflammation and inflammatory responses under control.

The above mentioned benefits are noticeable once the patient follows the diet for at least a month and then continuing it for longer periods, to avoid the stage where dialysis is needed. The strictness of the diet depends on the current stage of renal/kidney disease, if, for example, you are in the 3rd or 4th stage, you should follow a stricter diet and be attentive for the food, which is allowed or prohibited.

These exact foods and nutrients that you should take when following a renal diet, will be given to you in the following sections, and so keep on reading.

Explanation of key diet words

The following nutrients play a major role in a renal diet as some have the ability to improve the condition while others can make it worse. Essentially, renal diet is based on low consumption of certain nutrients like potassium and phosphorus simply because it promotes fluid buildup within the system of a kidney patient. Here is a brief explanation of the function of each nutrient and its role in a renal diet:

Potassium.

Potassium is a mineral that naturally occurs in certain foods and plays a role in regulating heart rhythm and muscle movement. It is also needed for keeping fluid and electrolyte balance in normal levels. Our kidneys keep only the right levels of potassium in our system, and when it is excess, they expel it via the urine.

The problem is, once kidneys can't function properly, all this excess potassium can't be expelled out and spikes up, causing symptoms like muscle and bone weakness, abnormal heartbeat, and heart failure in extreme cases.

Thus, a diet low in potassium is recommended to prevent buildup and avoid such negative side effects.

Sodium.

Sodium is a trace mineral that is found in most foods that we eat today and it is the key component of salt, which is actually a sodium compound mixed with chloride. Most food that we consume and especially processed food is highly loaded with salt, however, we may be eating sodium in other forms too e.g. fish. The key role of sodium is to regulate blood pressure, help regulate nerve function, and maintain the balance of acids in the blood. However, when sodium is excessively high and the kidneys can expel it, it can lead to the following symptoms: an elevated feeling of thirst, swelling of hands, feet and the face, elevated blood pressure, and problems with breathing.

This is why it is suggested to keep sodium intake low, to avoid the above.

Phosphorus.

Phosphorus is an essential mineral that is responsible for the development and regeneration of our bones. Phosphorus also plays a key role in the growth of connective tissue e.g. muscles and the regulation of muscle motions. When food we take contains phosphorus, it gets absorbed by the intestines and then gets deposited in our bones.

However, when kidneys are damaged or dysfunctioning, the excess phosphorus can't be expelled through our systems and causes problems such as: extracting calcium out of the bones/making them weaker, and leading to excess calcium in the bloodstream which interferes with blood vessels, heart, eye, and lung function.

Protein.

Protein is a nutritional compound that consists of amino acids, which play a key role in various system functions like cell communication, oxygen supply, and cellular metabolism. They are also a part of a healthy immune system.

Normally, Protein is not an issue for our kidneys. When Protein is metabolized, waste by-products are also created and are filtered through the kidneys. This waste along with extra renal proteins after will be expelled through urine.

However, when kidneys are unable to filter out excess Protein, it gets accumulated in the blood and cause problems.

This doesn't mean that renal disease patients should avoid Protein totally as it is still necessary for some metabolic functions, as long as it's taken in moderate amounts and based on the stage of renal disease.

Carbs.

Carbs act as a key source of fuel for our bodies. The consumption of carbs is turned into glucose in our system, which is a primary source of energy.

Carbs are ok to be eaten in moderation by kidney patients and the daily recommended allowance is up to 150 grams/day. However, patients that also have Diabetes (besides renal disease) should control their carb consumption to avoid any sudden spikes in their blood glucose.

Fat.

Being in balanced amounts, fats in our bodies act as an energy source, aid in the release of hormones, and help regulate blood pressure. They also carry some vitamins that are Fat-soluble such as A, D, E, and K, which are also very important for our systems. Not all fats are created equal still, few are good for our health and some are bad. Bad fats are saturated and Trans fats and are found in processed meat, dairy, and other products. They are also found in margarine and vegetable Fat shortenings.

Fat, in general, don't pose a risk for renal disease patients, however, it is suggested to limit the consumption of saturated and Tran's fats to avoid any cardiovascular problems e.g. elevated blood pressure and clogging of the arteries.

Dietary Fiber.

Dietary Fiber is a compound that can't be digested on its own by enzymes and acids in our stomach and intestines, but is needed for the system to aid in the digestion of our food and encourage bowel movements. They generally promote bowel regularity and decrease the likelihood of developing constipation inside the colon. Dietary Fiber is typically found in fruits, vegetables, seeds and whole grains.

In patients with renal disease, dietary Fiber is ok up to 28 grams/day as long as these plant foods don't contain high amounts of phosphorus or potassium.

Vitamins.

According to medical and dietary guidelines, our bodies need close to 13 vitamins to functions. Vitamins play a key role in metabolic functions and the normal functioning of our cardiovascular, digestive, nervous system and immune systems. The adoption of a nutritionally dense and balanced diet is necessary for getting all the vitamins our system needs. However, due to some diet restrictions e.g. sodium, many renal patients are in need of water-soluble vitamins like B-complex (B1, B2, B6, B12, folic acid, biotin) and small amounts of Vitamin C.

Minerals.

Minerals are needed for our system to maintain healthy connective tissue e.g. bones, muscles, and skin and facilitate the normal function of our hearts and central nervous systems.

Our kidneys typically expel any excess amount of minerals through our urine as some can lead to health symptoms e.g. muscle spasms when their levels are abnormally high.

However, as it was mentioned earlier, some minerals like potassium and phosphorus cannot be expelled by our kidneys when in excess and so their intake through diet should be limited.

Other trace minerals are perfectly fine when following a renal diet: iron, copper, zinc and selenium. A lack of these can lead to increased oxidative stress and thus, it is important to take sufficient amounts through diet or supplementation.

Fluids.

Fluids are necessary for the proper hydration of our systems in fact; lack of fluids can lead to dehydration and death in extreme cases.

However, in patients with renal dysfunction, fluids can quickly build up to the point of placing pressure to vital organs like the lungs and heart and becoming dangerous. This is the reason why many physicians advise their kidney patients to limit the consumption of fluids, especially during the last stages of the disorder.

Managing Kidney Disease through Diet

Patients who struggle from kidney health issues, going through kidney dialysis and have renal impairments need to not only go through medical treatment but also change their eating habit, lifestyle to make the situation better. Numerous researches have been finished on this, and the conclusion is food has a lot to do with how your kidney functions and its overall health.

The first thing to changing your lifestyle is knowing about how your kidney functions and how different food can trigger different reactions in the kidney function. There are certain nutrients that affect your kidney directly. Nutrients like sodium, Protein, phosphate, and potassium are the risky ones. You do not have to omit them altogether from your diet, but you need to limit or minimize their intake as much as possible. You cannot leave out essential nutrient like Protein from your diet, but you need to count how much Protein you are having per day. This is essential in order to keep balance in your muscles and maintaining a good functioning kidney.

A vast change in kidney patients is measuring how much fluid they are drinking. This is a crucial change in every kidney patient, and you must adapt to this new eating habit. Too much water or any other form of liquid can disrupt your kidney function. How much fluid you can consume depends on the condition of your kidney. Most people assign separate bottles for them so that they can measure how much they have drunk and how much more they can drink throughout the day.

What You Can and Can't Eat

Food to Eat

The renal diet aims to cut down the amount of waste in the blood. When people have kidney dysfunction, the kidneys are unable to remove and filter waste properly. When waste is left in the blood, it can affect the electrolyte levels of the patient. With a kidney diet, kidney function is promoted, and the progression of complete kidney failure is slowed down.

The renal diet follows a low intake of Protein, phosphorus, and sodium. It is necessary to consume high-quality Protein and limit some fluids. For some people, it is important to limit calcium and potassium.

Promoting a renal diet, here are the substances which are critical to be monitored:

Sodium and its role in the body

Most natural foods contain sodium. Some people think that sodium and salt are interchangeable. However, salt is a compound of chloride and sodium. There might be either salt or sodium in other forms in the food we eat. Due to the added salt, processed foods include a higher level of sodium.

Apart from potassium and chloride, sodium is one of the most crucial body's electrolytes. The main function of electrolytes is to control the fluids when they are going out and in the body's cells and tissues.

With sodium:

Blood volume and pressure are regulated.

Muscle contraction and nerve function are regulated.

The acid-base balance of the blood is regulated.

The amount of fluid the body eliminates and keeps is balanced.

Why is it important to monitor sodium intake for people with kidney issues?

Since the kidneys of kidney disease patients are unable to reduce excess fluid and sodium from the body adequately, too much sodium might be harmful. As fluid and sodium build up in the bloodstream and tissues, they might cause:

Edema: swelling in face, hands, and legs

Increased thirst

High blood pressure

Shortness of breath

Heart failure

The ways to monitor sodium intake:

Avoid processed foods

Be attentive to serving sizes.

Read food labels

Utilize fresh meats instead of processed

Choose fresh fruits and veggies.

Compare brands, choosing the ones with the lowest sodium levels.

Utilize spices that do not include salt

Ensure the sodium content is less than 400 mg per meal and not more than 150 mg per snack

Cook at home, not adding salt

Foods to eat with lower sodium content:

Fresh meats, dairy products, frozen veggies, and fruits

Fresh herbs and seasonings like rosemary, oregano, dill, lime, cilantro, onion, lemon, and garlic

Corn tortilla chips, pretzels, no salt added crackers, unsalted popcorn

Potassium and its role in the body

The main function of potassium is keeping muscles working correctly and the heartbeat regular. This mineral is responsible for maintaining electrolyte and fluid balance in the bloodstream. The kidneys regulate the proper amount of potassium in the body, expelling excess amounts in the urine.

Monitoring potassium intake

Limit high potassium food

Select only fresh fruits and veggies

Limit dairy products and milk to 8 oz. per day

Avoid potassium chloride

Read labels on packaged foods.

Avoid seasonings and salt substitutes with potassium.

Foods to eat with lower potassium:

Fruits: watermelon, tangerines, pineapple, plums, peaches, pears, papayas, mangoes, lemons and limes, honeydew, grapefruit/grapefruit juice, grapes/grape juice, clementine/satsuma, cranberry juice, berries, and apples/ applesauce, apple juice

Veggies: summer squash (cooked), okra, mushrooms (fresh), lettuce, kale, green beans, eggplant, cucumber, corn, onions (raw), celery, cauliflower, carrots, cabbage, broccoli (fresh), bamboo shoots (canned), and bell peppers

Plain Turkish delights, marshmallows and jellies, boiled fruit sweets, and peppermints

Shortbread, ginger nut biscuits, plain digestives

Plain flapjacks and cereal bars

Plain sponge cakes like Madeira cake, lemon sponge, jam sponge

Corn-based and wheat crisps

Whole grain crispbreads and crackers

Protein and other foods (bread (not whole grain), pasta, noodles, rice, eggs, canned tuna, turkey (white meat), and chicken (white meat)

Phosphorus and its role in the body

This mineral is essential in bone development and maintenance. Phosphorus helps in the development of connective organs and tissue and assists in muscle movement. Extra phosphorus is possible to be removed by healthy kidneys. However, it is impossible with kidney dysfunction. High levels of phosphorus make bones weak by pulling calcium out of your bones. It might lead to dangerous calcium deposits in the heart, eyes, lungs, and blood vessels.

Monitoring phosphorus intake

Pay attention to serving size

Eat fresh fruits and veggies

Eat smaller portions of foods that are rich in Protein

Avoid packaged foods

Keep a food journal

Foods to eat with low phosphorus level:

Grapes, apples

Lettuce, leeks

Carbs (white rice, corn, and rice Cereal, popcorn, pasta, crackers (not wheat), white bread)

Meat (sausage, fresh meat)

Protein

Damaged kidneys are unable to remove Protein waste, so they accumulate in the blood. The amount of Protein to consume differs depending on the stage of CKD. Protein is critical for tissue maintenance, and it is necessary to eat the proper amount of it according to the particular stage of kidneys disease.

Sources of Protein for vegetarians:

Vegans (allowing only plant-based foods): Wheat Protein and whole grains, nut butter, soy Protein, yogurt or soy milk, cooked no salt added canned and dried beans and peas, unsalted nuts.

Lacto vegetarians (allowing dairy products, milk, and plant-based foods): reduced-sodium or low-sodium cottage cheese.

Lacto-Ovo vegetarians (allowing eggs, dairy products, milk, and plant-based foods): eggs.

Food to Avoid

Food with high sodium content:

Onion salt, marinades, garlic salt, teriyaki sauce, and table salt

Pepperoni, bacon, ham, lunch meat, hot dogs, sausage, processed meats

Ramen noodles, canned produce, and canned soups

Marinara sauce, gravy, salad dressings, soy sauce, BBQ sauce, and ketchup

Chex Mix, salted nuts, Cheetos, crackers, and potato chips

Fast food

Food with a high potassium level:

Fruits: dried fruit, oranges/orange juice, prunes/prune juice, kiwi, nectarines, dates, cantaloupe, bananas, black currants, damsons, cherries, grapes, and apricots.

Vegetables: tomatoes/tomato sauce/tomato juice, sweet potatoes, beans, lentils, split peas, spinach (cooked), pumpkin, potatoes, mushrooms (cooked), chile peppers, chard, Brussels sprouts (cooked), broccoli (cooked), baked beans, avocado, butternut squash, and acorn squash.

Protein and other foods: peanut butter, molasses, granola, chocolate, bran, sardines, fish, bacon, ham, nuts and seeds, yogurt, milkshakes, and milk.

Coconut-based snacks, nut-based snacks, fudge, and toffee

Cakes containing marzipan.

Potato crisps.

Foods with high phosphorus:

Dairy products: pudding, ice cream, yogurt, cottage cheese, cheese, and milk

Nuts and seeds: sunflower seeds, pumpkin seeds, pecans, peanut butter, pistachios, cashews, and almonds

Dried beans and peas: soybeans, split peas, refried beans, pinto beans, lentils, kidney beans, garbanzo beans, black beans, and baked beans.

Meat: veal, turkey, liver, lamb, beef, bacon, fish, and seafood.

Carbs: whole grain products, oatmeal, and bran cereals

Chapter 1. Renal Diet Breakfast Recipes

1. Very Berry Smoothie

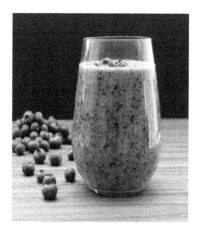

Preparation Time: 3 minutes

Cooking Time: 5 minutes

Servings: 2

Ingredients:

- 2 quarts water
- 2 cups pomegranate seeds
- 1 cup blackberries
- 1 cup blueberries

Directions:

1. Mix all ingredients in a blender.
2. Puree until smooth and creamy.
3. Transfer to a serving glass and enjoy.

Nutrition:

Calories: 464;

Carbs: 111g;

Protein: 8g;

Fat: 4g;

Phosphorus: 132mg;

Potassium: 843mg;

Sodium: 16mg

2. Pasta with Indian Lentils

Preparation Time: 5 minutes

Cooking Time: 0 minutes

Servings: 6

Ingredients:

- 1/4-1/2 cup fresh cilantro (chopped)
- 3 cups water
- 2 small dry red peppers (whole)
- 1 teaspoon turmeric
- 1 teaspoon ground cumin
- 2-3 cloves garlic (minced)
- 1 can (15 ounces) cubed tomatoes (with juice)
- 1 large onion (chopped)
- 1/2 cup dry lentils (rinsed)
- 1/2 cup orzo or tiny pasta

Directions:

1. In a skillet, combine ingredients except for the cilantro then boil on medium-high heat.
2. Ensure to cover and slightly reduce heat to medium-low and simmer until pasta is tender for about 35 minutes.
3. Afterwards, take out the chili peppers then add cilantro and top it with low-Fat sour cream.

Nutrition:

Calories: 175;

Carbs: 40g;

Protein: 3g;

Fat: 2g;

Phosphorus: 139mg;

Potassium: 513mg;

Sodium: 61mg

3. Pineapple Bread

Preparation Time: 20 Minutes

Cooking Time: 1 Hour

Servings: 10

Ingredients:

- 1/3 cup Swerve
- 1/3 cup butter, unsalted
- 2 eggs
- 2 cups flour
- 3 teaspoons baking powder
- 1 cup pineapple, undrained
- 6 cherries, chopped

Directions:

1. Whisk the Swerve with the butter in a mixer until fluffy.
2. Stir in the eggs, then beat again.
3. Add the baking powder and flour, then mix well until smooth.
4. Fold in the cherries and pineapple.
5. Spread this cherry-pineapple batter in a 9x5 inch baking pan.
6. Bake the pineapple batter for 1 hour at 350 degrees F.
7. Slice the bread and serve.

Nutrition:

Calories 197,

Total Fat 7.2g,

Sodium 85mg,

Dietary Fiber 1.1g,

Carbs 23.19 g,

Sugars 3 g,

Protein 4g,

Calcium 79mg,

Phosphorus 316mg,

Potassium 227mg

4. Parmesan Zucchini Frittata

Preparation Time: 10 minutes

Cooking Time: 35 minutes

Servings: 6

Ingredients:

- 1 tablespoon olive oil
- 1 cup yellow onion, sliced
- 3 cups zucchini, chopped
- 1/2 cup Parmesan cheese, grated
- 8 large eggs
- 1/2 teaspoon black pepper
- 1/8 teaspoon paprika
- 3 tablespoons parsley, chopped

Directions:

1. Toss the zucchinis with the onion, parsley, and all other ingredients in a large bowl.
2. Pour this zucchini-garlic mixture in an 11x7 inches pan and spread it evenly.
3. Bake the zucchini casserole for approximately 35 minutes at 350 degrees F.
4. Cut in slices and serve.

Nutrition:

Calories 142,

Total Fat 9.7g,

Saturated Fat 2.8g,

Cholesterol 250mg,

Sodium 123mg,

Carbs 4.7g,

Dietary Fiber 1.3g,

Sugars 2.4g,

Protein 10.2g,

Calcium 73mg,

Phosphorus 375mg,

Potassium 286mg

5. Texas Toast Casserole

Preparation Time: 10 minutes

Cooking Time: 30 minutes

Servings: 10

Ingredients:

- 1/2 cup butter, melted
- 1 cup brown Swerve
- 1 lb. Texas Toast bread, sliced
- 4 large eggs
- 1 1/2 cup milk
- 1 tablespoon vanilla extract
- 2 tablespoons Swerve
- 2 teaspoons cinnamon
- Maple syrup for serving

Directions:

1. Layer a 9x13 inches baking pan with cooking spray.
2. Spread the bread slices at the bottom of the prepared pan.
3. Whisk the eggs with the remaining ingredients in a mixer.
4. Pour this mixture over the bread slices evenly.
5. Bake the bread for 30 minutes at 350 degrees F in a preheated oven.
6. Serve.

Nutrition:

Calories 332,

Total Fat 13.7g,

Sodium 350mg,

Dietary Fiber 2g,

Sugars 6g,

Carbs 47.11 g,

Protein 7.4g,

Calcium 143mg,

Phosphorus 186mg,

Potassium 74mg

6. Garlic Mayo Bread

Preparation Time: 10 minutes

Cooking Time: 5 minutes

Servings: 16

Ingredients:

- 3 tablespoons vegetable oil
- 4 cloves garlic, minced
- 2 teaspoons paprika
- Dash cayenne pepper
- 1 teaspoon lemon juice
- 2 tablespoons Parmesan cheese, grated
- 3/4 cup mayonnaise
- 1 loaf (1 lb.) French bread, sliced
- 1 teaspoon Italian herbs

Directions:

1. Mix the garlic with the oil in a small bowl and leave it overnight.
2. Discard the garlic from the bowl and keep the garlic-infused oil.
3. Mix the garlic-oil with cayenne, paprika, lemon juice, mayonnaise, and Parmesan.
4. Place the bread slices in a baking tray lined with parchment paper.
5. Top these slices with the mayonnaise mixture and drizzle the Italian herbs on top.
6. Broil these slices for 5 minutes until golden brown.

7. Serve warm.

Nutrition:

Calories 217,

Total Fat 7.9g,

Sodium 423mg,

Dietary Fiber 1.3g,

Sugars 2g,

Carbs 5.36 g,

Protein 7g,

Calcium 56mg,

Phosphorus 347mg,

Potassium 72mg

7. Strawberry Topped Waffles

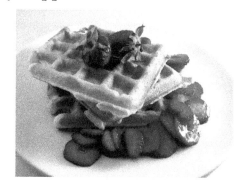

Preparation Time: 15 minutes

Cooking Time: 20 minutes

Servings: 5

Ingredients:

- 1 cup flour
- 1/4 cup Swerve
- 1 3/4 teaspoons baking powder
- 1 egg, separated
- 3/4 cup milk
- 1/2 cup butter, melted
- 1/2 teaspoon vanilla extract
- Fresh strawberries, sliced

Directions:

1. Prepare and preheat your waffle pan following the instructions of the machine.
2. Begin by mixing the flour with Swerve and baking soda in a bowl.

3. Separate the egg yolks from the egg whites, keeping them in two separate bowls.
4. Add the milk and vanilla extract to the egg yolks.
5. Stir the melted butter and mix well until smooth.
6. Now beat the egg whites with an electric beater until foamy and fluffy.
7. Fold this fluffy composition in the egg yolk mixture.
8. Mix it gently until smooth, then add in the flour mixture.
9. Stir again to make a smooth mixture.
10. Pour a half cup of the waffle batter in a preheated pan and cook until the waffle is done.
11. Cook more waffles with the remaining batter.
12. Serve fresh with strawberries on top.

Nutrition:

Calories 342,

Total Fat 20.5g,

Sodium 156mg,

Dietary Fiber 0.7g,

Sugars 3.5g,

Carbs 21.28 g,

Protein 4.8g,

Calcium 107mg,

Phosphorus 126mg,

Potassium 233mg

8. Cheese Spaghetti Frittata

Preparation Time: 10 minutes

Cooking Time: 10 minutes

Servings: 6

Ingredients:

- 4 cups whole-wheat spaghetti, cooked
- 4 teaspoons olive oil
- 3 medium onions, chopped
- 4 large eggs
- 1/2 cup milk
- 1/3 cup Parmesan cheese, grated
- 2 tablespoons fresh parsley, chopped
- 2 tablespoons fresh basil, chopped
- 1/2 teaspoon black pepper
- 1 tomato, diced

Directions:

1. Set a suitable non-stick skillet over moderate heat and add in the olive oil.
2. Place the spaghetti in the skillet and cook by stirring for 2 minutes on moderate heat.
3. Whisk the eggs with milk, parsley, and black pepper in a bowl.
4. Pour this milky egg mixture over the spaghetti and top it all with basil, cheese, and tomato.
5. Cover the spaghetti frittata again with a lid and cook for approximately 8 minutes on low heat.
6. Slice and serve.

Nutrition:

Calories 230,

Total Fat 7.8g,

Sodium 77mg,

Dietary Fiber 5.6g,

Sugars 4.5g,

Carbs 198.36 g

Protein 11.1g,

Calcium 88mg,

Phosphorus 368 mg,

Potassium 214mg,

9. Shrimp Bruschetta

Preparation Time: 15 minutes

Cooking Time: 10 minutes

Servings: 4

Ingredients:

- 13 oz. shrimps, peeled
- 1 tablespoon tomato sauce
- 1/2 teaspoon Splenda
- 1/4 teaspoon garlic powder
- 1 teaspoon fresh parsley, chopped
- 1/2 teaspoon olive oil
- 1 teaspoon lemon juice
- 4 whole-grain bread slices
- 1 cup water, for cooking

Directions:

1. In the saucepan, pour water and bring it to boil.
2. Add shrimps and boil them over the high heat for 5 minutes.
3. After this, drain shrimps and chill them to the room temperature.
4. Mix up together shrimps with Splenda, garlic powder, tomato sauce, and fresh parsley.
5. Add lemon juice and stir gently.
6. Heat an oven to 360f.
7. Coat the slice of bread with olive oil and bake for 3 minutes.

8. Then place the shrimp mixture on the bread. Bruschetta is cooked.

Nutrition:

Calories 199,

Fat 3.7,

Fiber 2.1,

Carbs 15.3,

Protein 24.1

Phosphorus 294 mg

Potassium 359 mg

Sodium 325 mg

10. Strawberry Muesli

Preparation Time: 10 minutes

Cooking Time: 30 minutes

Servings: 4

Ingredients:

- 2 cups Greek yogurt
- 1 1/2 cup strawberries, sliced
- 1 1/2 cup Muesli
- 4 teaspoon maple syrup
- 3/4 teaspoon ground cinnamon

Directions:

1. Put Greek yogurt in the food processor.
2. Add 1 cup of strawberries, maple syrup, and ground cinnamon.
3. Blend the ingredients until you get smooth mass.
4. Transfer the yogurt mass in the serving bowls.
5. Add Muesli and stir well.
6. Leave the meal for 30 minutes in the fridge.
7. After this, decorate it with remaining sliced strawberries.

Nutrition:

Calories 149,

Fat 2.6,

Fiber 3.6,

Carbs 21.6,

Protein 12

Phosphorus 130 mg

Potassium 289 mg

Sodium 58 mg

11. Yogurt Bulgur

Preparation Time: 10 minutes

Cooking Time: 15 minutes

Servings: 3

Ingredients:

- 1 cup bulgur
- 2 cups Greek yogurt
- 1 1/2 cup water
- 1/2 teaspoon salt
- 1 teaspoon olive oil

Directions:

1. Pour olive oil in the saucepan and add bulgur.
2. Roast it over the medium heat for 2-3 minutes. Stir it from time to time.
3. After this, add salt and water.
4. Close the lid and cook bulgur for 15 minutes over the medium heat.
5. Then chill the cooked bulgur well and combine it with Greek yogurt. Stir it carefully.
6. Transfer the cooked meal into the serving plates. The yogurt bulgur tastes the best when it is cold.

Nutrition:

Calories 274,

Fat 4.9,

Fiber 8.5,

Carbs 40.8,

Protein 19.2

Phosphorus 179 mg

Potassium 295 mg

Sodium 468 mg

12. Sun-Dried Tomato Frittata

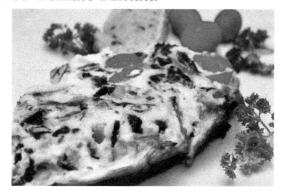

Preparation Time: 10 minutes

Cooking Time: 20 minutes

Servings: 8

Ingredients:

- 12 eggs
- 1/2 tsp dried basil
- 1/4 cup parmesan cheese, grated
- 2 cups baby spinach, shredded
- 1/4 cup sun-dried tomatoes, sliced
- Pepper
- Salt

Directions:

1. Heat an oven to 425 F. In a large bowl, whisk eggs with pepper and salt.
2. Add remaining ingredients and stir to combine. Spray oven-safe pan with cooking spray.
3. Pour egg mixture into the pan and bake for 20 minutes.
4. Slice and serve.

Nutrition:

Calories 115

Fat 7g

Carbs 1g

Sugar 1g

Carbs 3.73 g

Phosphorus 263 mg

Potassium 359 mg

Sodium 220 mg

Protein 10g

Cholesterol 250 mg

13. Italian Breakfast Frittata

Preparation Time: 10 minutes

Cooking Time: 45 minutes

Servings: 4

Ingredients:

- 2 cups egg whites
- 1/2 cup mozzarella cheese, shredded
- 1 cup cottage cheese, crumbled
- 1/4 cup fresh basil, sliced
- 1/2 cup roasted red peppers, sliced
- Pepper
- Salt

Directions:

1. Heat an oven to 375 F.
2. Add all ingredients into large bowl and whisk well to combine.
3. Pour frittata mixture into the baking dish and bake for 45 minutes.
4. Slice and serve.

Nutrition:

Calories 131

Fat 2g

Carbs 5g

Carbs 5.39 g

Phosphorus 203 mg

Potassium 338 mg

Sodium 499 mg

Sugar 2g

Protein 22g

Cholesterol 6mg

14. Greek Egg Scrambled

Preparation Time: 10 minutes

Cooking Time: 10 minutes

Servings: 2

Ingredients:

- 4 eggs
- 1/2 cup grape tomatoes, sliced
- 2 tbsp. green onions, sliced
- 1 bell pepper, diced
- 1 tbsp. olive oil
- 1/4 tsp dried oregano
- 1/2 tbsp. capers
- 3 olives, sliced
- Pepper
- Salt

Directions:

1. Heat an oil in pan over medium heat
2. Add green onions and bell pepper and cook until pepper is softened.
3. Add tomatoes, capers, and olives and cook for 1 minute.
4. Add eggs and stir until eggs are cooked. Season it with oregano, pepper, and salt.
5. Serve and enjoy.

Nutrition:

Calories 230

Fat 17g

Carbs 8g

Carbs 13.83 g

Phosphorus 338 mg

Potassium 550 mg

Sodium 323 mg

Sugar 5g

Protein 12g

Cholesterol 325 mg

15. Feta Mint Omelet

Preparation Time: 10 minutes

Cooking Time: 5 minutes

Servings: 1

Ingredients:

- 3 eggs
- 1/4 cup fresh mint, chopped
- 2 tbsp. coconut milk
- 1/2 tsp olive oil
- 2 tbsp. feta cheese, crumbled
- Pepper
- Salt

Directions:

1. In a bowl, whisk eggs with feta cheese, mint, milk, pepper, and salt.
2. Heat olive oil in a pan over low heat. Pour egg mixture in the pan and cook until eggs are set.
3. Flip omelet and cook for 2 minutes more.
4. Serve and enjoy.

Nutrition:

Calories 275

Fat 20g

Carbs 4g

Carbs 11.4 g

Phosphorus 861 mg

Potassium 868 mg

Sodium 840 mg

Sugar 2g

Protein 20g

Cholesterol 505 mg

16. Sausage Breakfast Casserole

Preparation Time: 10 minutes

Cooking Time: 50 minutes

Servings: 8

Ingredients:

- 12 eggs
- 1 lb. ground Italian sausage
- 2 1/2 tomatoes, sliced
- 3 tbsp. coconut flour
- 1/4 cup coconut milk
- 2 small zucchinis, shredded
- Pepper
- Salt

Directions:

1. Heat an oven to 350 F.
2. Spray casserole dish w/ cooking spray and set aside.
3. Cook sausage in a pan until brown.
4. Transfer sausage to a mixing bowl.
5. Add coconut flour, milk, eggs, zucchini, pepper, and salt. Stir well.
6. Add eggs and whisk to combine.
7. Transfer bowl mixture into the casserole dish and top with tomato slices.
8. Bake for 50 minutes.
9. Serve and enjoy.

Nutrition:

Calories 305

Fat 21.8g

Carbs 6.3g

Carbs 3.26 g

Phosphorus 325 mg

Potassium 444 mg

Sodium 578 mg

Sugar 3.3g

Protein 19.6g

Cholesterol 286 mg

17. Easy Turnip Puree

Preparation Time: 10 minutes

Cooking Time: 12 minutes

Servings: 4

Ingredients:

- 1 1/2 lbs. turnips, peeled and chopped
- 1 tsp dill
- 3 bacon slices, cooked and chopped
- 2 tbsp. fresh chives, chopped

Directions:

1. Add turnip into the boiling water and cook for 12 minutes. Drain well and place in a food processor.
2. Add dill and process until smooth.
3. Transfer turnip puree into the bowl and top with bacon and chives.
4. Serve and enjoy.

Nutrition:

Calories 127

Fat 6g

Carbs 11.6g

Carbs 8.48 g

Phosphorus 90 mg

Potassium 471 mg

Sodium 124 mg

Sugar 7g

Protein 6.8g

Cholesterol 16 mg

18. Spinach Bacon Breakfast Bake

Preparation Time: 10 minutes

Cooking Time: 45 minutes

Servings: 6

Ingredients:

- 10 eggs
- 3 cups baby spinach, chopped
- 1 tbsp. olive oil
- 8 bacon slices, cooked and chopped
- 2 tomatoes, sliced
- 2 tbsp. chives, chopped
- Pepper
- Salt

Directions:

1. Heat an oven to 350 F.
2. Spray a baking dish w/ cooking spray and set aside.
3. Heat an oil in pan
4. Add spinach and cook until spinach wilted.
5. In a mixing bowl, whisk eggs and salt. Add spinach and chives and stir well.
6. Pour egg mixture into the baking dish.
7. Top with tomatoes and bacon and bake for 45 minutes.
8. Serve and enjoy.

Nutrition:

Calories 273

Fat 20.4g

Carbs 3.1g

Carbs 3.47 g

Phosphorus 332 mg

Potassium 558 mg

Sodium 346 mg

Sugar 1.7g

Protein 19.4g

Cholesterol 301 mg

19. Healthy Spinach Tomato Muffins

Preparation Time: 10 minutes

Cooking Time: 20 minutes

Servings: 12

Ingredients:

- 12 eggs
- 1/2 tsp Italian seasoning
- 1 cup tomatoes, chopped
- 4 tbsp. water
- 1 cup fresh spinach, chopped
- Pepper
- Salt

Directions:

1. Heat an oven to 350 F. Spray a muffin tray with cooking spray and set aside.
2. In a mixing bowl, whisk eggs with water, Italian seasoning, pepper, and salt.
3. Add spinach and tomatoes and stir well.
4. Pour egg mixture into the prepared muffin tray and bake for 20 minutes.
5. Serve and enjoy.

Nutrition:
Calories 67

Fat 4.5g

Carbs 1g

Carbs 2.01 g

Phosphorus 160 mg

Potassium 213 mg

Sodium 114 mg

Sugar 0.8g

Protein 5.7g

Cholesterol 164 mg

20. Chicken Egg Breakfast Muffins

Preparation Time: 10 minutes

Cooking Time: 15 minutes

Servings: 12

Ingredients:

- 10 eggs
- 1 cup cooked chicken, chopped
- 3 tbsp. green onions, chopped
- 1/4 tsp garlic powder
- Pepper
- Salt

Directions:

1. Heat an oven to 400 F. Spray a muffin tray with cooking spray and set aside. In a large bowl, whisk eggs with garlic powder, pepper, and salt.
2. Add remaining ingredients and stir well. Pour egg mixture into the muffin tray and bake for 15 minutes. Serve and enjoy.

Nutrition:

Calories 71

Fat 4 g

Carbs 0.4g

Carbs 1.34 g

Phosphorus 142 mg

Potassium 158 mg

Sodium 92 mg

Sugar 0.3g

Protein 8g

Cholesterol 145 mg

21. Vegetable Tofu Scramble

Preparation Time: 10 minutes

Cooking Time: 7 minutes

Servings: 2

Ingredients:

- 1/2 block firm tofu, crumbled
- 1/4 tsp ground cumin
- 1 tbsp. turmeric
- 1 cup spinach
- 1/4 cup zucchini, chopped
- 1 tbsp. olive oil
- 1 tomato, chopped
- 1 tbsp. chives, chopped
- 1 tbsp. coriander, chopped
- Pepper
- Salt

Directions:

1. Heat an oil in pan over medium heat
2. Add tomato, zucchini, and spinach and sauté for 2 minutes.
3. Add tofu, cumin, turmeric, pepper, and salt and sauté for 5 minutes.
4. Top with chives, and coriander.
5. Serve and enjoy.

Nutrition:

Calories 101

Fat 8.5 g

Carbs 5.1g

Carbs 11.92 g

Phosphorus 204 mg

Potassium 614 mg

Sodium 30 mg

Sugar 1.4g

Protein 3.1g

Cholesterol 0 mg

22. Keto Overnight Oats

Preparation Time: 5 minutes

Cooking Time: 5 minutes

Servings: 2

Ingredients:

- 1 tbsp. chia seed
- 4 drops liquid stevia
- 1/2 cup hemp hearts
- 2/3 cup coconut milk
- 1/2 tsp vanilla
- Pinch of salt

Directions:

1. Add all ingredients into bowl & mix well.
2. Cover then put it in the refrigerator for 8 hours.
3. Serve and enjoy.

Nutrition:

Calories 289

Fat 22.5g

Carbs 5g

Carbs 5.73 g

Phosphorus 92 mg

Potassium 174 mg

Sodium 191 mg

Sugar 0.1g

Protein 14g

Cholesterol 0 mg

23. Cheese Coconut Pancakes

Preparation Time: 10 minutes

Cooking Time: 5 minutes

Servings: 1

Ingredients:

- 2 eggs
- 1 packet stevia
- 1/2 tsp cinnamon
- 2 oz. cream cheese
- 1 tbsp. coconut flour
- 1/2 tsp vanilla

Directions:

1. Add all ingredients into bowl and blend until smooth.
2. Spray pan with cooking spray and heat over medium-high heat.
3. Pour batter on the hot pan and make two pancakes.
4. Cook pancake until lightly brown from both the sides.
5. Serve and enjoy.

Nutrition:

Calories 386

Fat 30g

Carbs 12g

Carbs 5.88 g

Phosphorus 364 mg

Potassium 421 mg

Sodium 468 mg

Sugar 1g

Protein 16g

Cholesterol 389 mg

24. Coconut Breakfast Smoothie

Preparation Time: 5 minutes

Cooking Time: 5 minutes

Servings: 1

Ingredients:

- 1/4 cup whey Protein powder
- 1/2 cup coconut milk
- 5 drops liquid stevia
- 1 tbsp. coconut oil
- 1 tsp vanilla
- 2 tbsp. coconut butter
- 1/4 cup water
- 1/2 cup ice

Directions:

1. Add all fixings into the blender then blend until smooth.
2. Serve and enjoy.

Nutrition:

Calories 560

Fat 45g

Carbs 12g

Carbs 6.38 g

Phosphorus 110 mg

Potassium 174 mg

Sodium 237 mg

Sugar 4g

Protein 25g

Cholesterol 60 mg

25. Cinnamon Cheese Pancakes

Preparation Time: 10 minutes

Cooking Time: 10 minutes

Servings: 4

Ingredients:

- 4 eggs
- 1/2 cup cream cheese
- 1/2 cup almond flour
- 1 tbsp. butter, melted
- 1/2 tsp cinnamon

Directions:

1. Add all ingredients except butter into the blender and blend until well combined.
2. The heat melted butter in a pan over medium heat.
3. Pour 3 tbsp. of batter on the pan and make pancakes and cook for 2 minutes on each side.
4. Serve and enjoy.

Nutrition:

Calories 271

Fat 24 g

Carbs 4g

Carbs 2.36 g

Phosphorus 183 mg

Potassium 192 mg

Sodium 256 mg

Sugar 1g

Protein 10g

Cholesterol 201 mg

26. Breakfast Egg Salad

Preparation Time: 10 minutes

Cooking Time: 5 minutes

Servings: 4

Ingredients:

- 6 eggs, hard-boiled, peeled and chopped
- 1/2 cup dill pickles, chopped
- 1 tbsp. fresh dill, chopped
- 4 tbsp. mayonnaise
- Pepper & Salt

Directions:

1. Add all ingredients into large bowl and stir to mix. Serve and enjoy.

Nutrition:

Calories 140

Fat 10g

Carbs 4g

Carbs 4.44 g

Phosphorus 249 mg

Potassium 314 mg

Sodium 458 mg

Sugar 1g

Protein 8g

Cholesterol 245 mg

27. Creamy Cinnamon Scrambled Egg

Preparation Time: 10 minutes

Cooking Time: 5 minutes

Servings: 2

Ingredients:

- 4 eggs
- 1/4 tsp ground cinnamon
- 2 tbsp. heavy cream
- 1 tbsp. butter
- Pepper
- Salt

Directions:

1. In a bowl, whisk together eggs & heavy cream.
2. Melt butter in a pan over medium heat.
3. Add the egg mixture in a pan and stir until eggs are cooked. Remove pan from heat.
4. Sprinkle with ground cinnamon.
5. Serve and enjoy.

Nutrition:

Calories 186

Fat 15g

Carbs 1g

Carbs 4.86 g

Phosphorus 330 mg

Potassium 402 mg

Sodium 257 mg

Sugar 1g

Protein 12g

Cholesterol 346 mg

28. Choco Coconut Smoothie

Preparation Time: 5 minutes

Cooking Time: 5 minutes

Servings: 1

Ingredients:

- 1/2 tbsp. cocoa powder
- 1/4 cup heavy cream
- 5 drops liquid stevia
- 1/4 cup coconut milk
- 1/2 cup unsweetened almond milk

Directions:

1. Add all ingredients to the blender & blend until smooth.
2. Serve and enjoy.

Nutrition:

Calories 201

Fat 19g

Carbs 7g

Carbs 11.16 g

Phosphorus 192 mg

Potassium 332 mg

Sodium 91 mg

Sugar 3g

Protein 2g

Cholesterol 10 mg

Chapter 2. Renal Diet Snacks Recipes

29. Ginger-Lime Grilled Shrimp

Preparation Time: 5 minutes

Cooking Time: 6 minutes

Servings: 3-4

Ingredients:

- 2 tbsp. lime juice;
- 1/4 tbsp. crushed red pepper flakes;
- 3 cloves garlic;
- 2 tsp freshly-grated ginger;
- 1/4 tsp salt;
- 1/4 tsp ground black pepper;
- 2 tbsp. fresh cilantro leaves;
- 1 tbsp. extra-virgin olive oil;
- 1-2 pounds large shrimp;

Directions:

1. Mince the garlic and cilantro leaves.
2. Mix lime juice, red pepper flakes, garlic, ginger, salt, black pepper, and cilantro in a bowl, and then drizzle in the oil, stirring constantly.
3. Pierce the shrimp at the head end & carefully cut along the back toward the tail, removing the dark vein.
4. Rinse in running water. Pat dry, and then place in a bowl and mix with the
5. Marinade well. Cover tightly and place into the fridge for 20 minutes.
6. Preheat the gas grill on high heat.

7. Thread the shrimp on skewers, leaving a little room between them. Grill for 2-3 minutes per side with the lid closed.

Nutrition:

Calories: 23.5

Fat: 13g

Carbs: 0.6g

Protein: 2g

Phosphorus

Potassium

Sodium

30. Seafood Jambalaya

Preparation Time: 20 minutes

Cooking Time: 25 minutes

Servings: 4

Ingredients:

- 1 lb. wild Alaskan cod fillets;
- 1 lb. shrimp;
- 2 cups chicken broth;
- 2 red bell peppers;
- 4-5 carrots;
- 1 leek;
- Sea salt to taste;
- 1 tbsp. chili powder;
- 1/2 tsp paprika;
- 1/2 tsp black pepper;
- 4 cloves garlic;
- 1/4 cup organic butter;
- Hot sauce to taste;

Directions:

1. Remove shrimp's tails and shells.
2. Slice the peppers and carrots. Dice leek, mince garlic.
3. Pat the fish and shrimp dry with a paper towel.
4. Cut the fish into medium pieces.
5. Melt butter in large soup pot, add carrots and stew for 4 minutes.
6. Add the bell peppers and garlic and cook for another 3-4 minutes.

7. Add all the spices and the chicken broth and bring to a boil.
8. Then add the fish and shrimp and simmer until the fish begins to flake and the shrimp turn pink and float.
9. Add the hot sauce and stir well.

Nutrition:

Calories: 207.6

Fat: 4.4g

Carbs: 30.1g

Protein: 11.6g

Phosphorus 948 mg

Potassium 1339 mg

Sodium 840 mg

31. Kale Chips

Preparation Time: 20 minutes

Cooking Time: 25 minutes

Servings: 6

Ingredients:

- 2 cups Kale
- 2 tsp of olive oil
- 1/4 tsp of chili powder
- Pinch cayenne pepper

Directions:

1. Heat an oven to 300F.
2. Line 2 baking sheets w/ parchment paper; set aside.
3. Remove the stems from the kale and tear the leaves into 2-inch pieces.
4. Wash the kale and dry it completely.
5. Transfer the kale to a large bowl and drizzle with olive oil.
6. Use your hands to toss the kale with oil, taking care to coat each leaf evenly.
7. Season the kale with chili powder and cayenne pepper and toss to combine thoroughly.
8. Spread the seasoned kale in a single layer on each baking sheet. Do not overlap the leaves.
9. Bake the kale, rotating the pans once, for 20 to 25 minutes until it is crisp and dry.
10. Remove the trays from oven and allow the chips to cool on the trays for 5 minutes.
11. Serve.

Nutrition:

Calories: 24

Fat: 2g

Carbs: 2g

Phosphorus: 21mg

Potassium: 111mg

Sodium: 13mg

Protein: 1g

32. Tortilla Chips

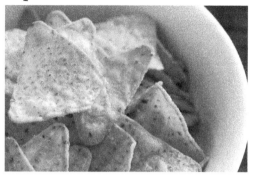

Preparation Time: 15 minutes

Cooking Time: 10 minutes

Servings: 6

Ingredients:

- 2 tsp granulated sugar
- 1/2 tsp ground cinnamon
- Pinch ground nutmeg
- Flour tortillas – 3 (6-inch)
- Cooking spray

Directions:

1. Heat an oven to 350F.
2. Line a baking sheet with parchment paper.
3. In a small bowl, stir the sugar, cinnamon, and nutmeg.
4. Lay the tortillas on a clean work surface and spray both sides of each lightly with cooking spray.
5. Sprinkle the cinnamon sugar evenly over both sides of each tortilla.

6. Cut the tortillas into 16 wedges each and place them on the baking sheet.
7. Bake the tortilla wedges, turning once, for about 10 minutes or until crisp.
8. Cool the chips serve.

Nutrition:

Calories: 51

Fat: 1g

Carbs: 9g

Phosphorus: 29mg

Potassium: 24mg

Sodium: 103mg

Protein: 1g

33. Baked Cream Cheese Crab Dip

Preparation Time: 5 minutes

Cooking Time: 30 minutes

Servings: 12

Ingredients:

- 8 oz. lump crab meat
- 8 oz. cream cheese softened
- 1/2 cup avocado mayonnaise
- 1 tablespoon lemon juice
- 1 teaspoon Worcestershire sauce
- 1/2 teaspoon of garlic powder
- 1/2 teaspoon of onion powder
- 1/2 teaspoon of salt
- 1/4 teaspoon of dry mustard
- 1/4 teaspoon of black pepper

Directions:

1. Add ingredients into small baking dish and spread out evenly. Bake at 375°F for about 25 to 30 minutes.
2. Serve with low carb crackers or vegetables. Enjoy.

Nutrition:

Calories: 167

Fat: 12g,

Carbs: 21g

Fiber: 2g

Protein: 31g

Phosphorus 143 mg

Potassium 420 mg

Sodium 188 mg

34. Herbal Cream Cheese Tartines

Preparation Time: 15 minutes

Cooking Time: 15 minutes

Servings: 2

Ingredients:

- 20 regular round melba crackers
- 1 clove garlic, halved
- 1 cup cream cheese spread
- 1/4 cup chopped herbs such as chives, dill, parsley, tarragon, or thyme
- 2 tbsp. minced French shallot or onion
- 1/2 tsp. black pepper
- 2 tbsp. tablespoons water

Directions:

1. In a medium-sized bowl, combine the cream cheese, herbs, shallot, pepper, and water with a hand blender.

2. Rub the crackers with the cut side of the garlic clove.

3. Serve the cream cheese with the rusks.

Nutrition:

Calories: 476

Fat: 9g

Carbs: 75g

Protein: 23g

Sodium: 885mg

Potassium: 312mg

Phosphorus: 165mg

35. Baba Ghanouj

Preparation Time: 10 minutes

Cooking Time: 1 hour and 20 minutes

Servings: 1

Ingredients:

- 1 large aubergine, cut in half lengthwise
- 1 head of garlic, unpeeled
- 30 ml (2 tablespoons) of olive oil
- Lemon juice to taste

Directions:

1. Heat an oven to 350 degrees F.

2. Place the eggplant on the plate, skin side up. Roast until the meat is very tender and detaches easily from the skin, about 1 hour depending on the eggplant's size. Let cool.

3. Meanwhile, cut the tip of the garlic cloves. Put garlic cloves in a square aluminum foil. Fold the edges of the sheet and fold together to form a tightly wrapped foil.

4. Roast with the eggplant until tender, about 20 minutes. Let cool. Purée the pods with a garlic press.

5. With a spoon, scoop out the eggplant's flesh and place it in the bowl of a food processor. Add the garlic puree, the oil, and the lemon juice. Stir until purée is smooth and pepper.

6. Serve with mini pita bread.

Nutrition:

Calories: 110

Fat: 12g

Carbs: 5g

Protein: 1g

Sodium: 180mg

Potassium: 207mg

Phosphorus: 81mg

36. Eggplant and Chickpea Bites

Preparation Time: 15 minutes

Cooking Time: 50 minutes

Servings: 6

Ingredients:

- 3 large aubergine cut in half (make a few cuts in the flesh with a knife)
- 2 large cloves garlic, peeled and deglazed
- 2 tbsp. coriander powder
- 2 tbsp. cumin seeds
- 400 g canned chickpeas, rinsed and drained
- 2 Tbsp. chickpea flour
- Zest and juice of 1/2 lemon
- 1/2 lemon quartered for serving
- 3 tbsp. tablespoon of polenta

Directions:

1. Heat the oven to 200°C. Spray the eggplant halves generously with oil and place them on the meat side up on a baking sheet.

2. Sprinkle with coriander and cumin seeds, and then place the cloves of garlic on the plate.

3. Season and roast for 40 minutes until the flesh of eggplant is completely tender. Reserve and let cool a little.

4. Scrape the flesh of the eggplant in a bowl with a spatula and throw the skins in the compost. Thoroughly scrape and make sure to incorporate spices and crushed roasted garlic.

5. Add chickpeas, chickpea flour, zest, and lemon juice. Crush roughly and mix well.

6. Check to season. Do not worry if the mixture seems a bit soft - it will firm up in the fridge.

7. Form about twenty pellets and place them on a baking sheet covered with parchment paper. Refrigerate for at least 30 minutes.

8. Heat up an oven to 180°C. Remove the meatballs from the fridge and coat them by rolling them in the polenta.

9. Place them back on the baking sheet and spray a little oil on each. Roast for 20 minutes until golden and crisp.

10. Serve with lemon wedges. You can also serve these dumplings with a spicy yogurt dip.

Nutrition:

Calories: 72

Fat: 1g

Carbs: 18g

Protein: 3g

Sodium: 63mg

Potassium: 162mg

Phosphorus: 36mg

37. Greek Cookies

Preparation Time: 20 minutes

Cooking Time: 25 minutes

Servings: 6

Ingredients:

- 1/2 cup Plain yogurt
- 1/2 teaspoon baking powder
- 2 tablespoons Erythritol
- 1 teaspoon almond extract
- 1/2 teaspoon ground clove
- 1/2 teaspoon orange zest, grated
- 3 tablespoons walnuts, chopped
- 1 cup wheat flour
- 1 teaspoon butter, softened
- 1 tablespoon honey
- 3 tablespoons water

Directions:

1. In the mixing bowl mix up together the plain yogurt, baking powder, Erythritol, almond extract, ground cloves orange zest, flour, and butter.
2. Knead the non-sticky dough. Add olive oil if the dough is very sticky and knead it well.
3. Then make the log from the dough and cut it into small pieces.
4. Roll every piece of dough into the balls and transfer in the lined with baking paper tray.
5. Press the balls gently and bake for 25 minutes at 350F.

6. Meanwhile, heat up together honey and water. Simmer the liquid for 1 minute and remove from the heat.
7. When the cookies are cooked, remove them from the oven and let them cool for 5 minutes.
8. Then pour the cookies with sweet honey water and sprinkle with walnuts.
9. Cool the cookies.

Nutrition:

Calories 134

Fat 3.4

Fiber 0.9

Carbs 26.1

Protein 4.3

Phosphorus 63 mg

Potassium 79 mg

Sodium 15 mg

38. Ham and Dill Pickle Bites

Preparation Time: 5 minutes

Cooking Time: 45 minutes

Servings: 6

Ingredients:

- Dill pickles
- Thin deli ham slices
- Cream cheese (or use whipped cream cheese if you prefer)

Directions:

1. Let the cream cheese sit for at least 30 minutes at room temperature before you make these. Cut dill pickles lengthwise into sixths, depending on how thick the pickles are. You need as many cut pickles spears as you have ham slices.
2. Spread each slice of ham with a very thin layer of cream cheese. Place a dill pickle on the edge of each ham slice. Then roll up the ham around the dill pickle, and place toothpicks where you want each piece to be cut. Arrange on plate and serve. Enjoy.

Nutrition:

Calories: 217

Fat: 11g

Carbs: 17g

Fiber: 6g

Protein: 20g

Phosphorus 4 mg

Potassium 26 mg

Sodium 182 mg

39. Easy Flavored Potatoes Mix

Preparation Time: 10 minutes

Cooking Time: 25 minutes

Servings: 2

Ingredients:

- 4 potatoes, thinly sliced
- 2 tablespoons olive oil
- 1 fennel bulb, thinly sliced
- 1 tablespoon dill, chopped
- 8 cherry tomatoes, halved
- Salt and black pepper to the taste

Directions:

1. Preheat an air fryer to 365 degrees F and add the oil.
2. Add potato slices, fennel, dill, tomatoes, salt and pepper, toss, cover and cook for 25 minutes.
3. Divide potato mix between plates and serve.
4. Enjoy!

Nutrition:

Calories 240

Fat 3

Fiber 2

Carbs 5

Protein 12

Phosphorus 490 mg

Potassium 3668 mg

Sodium 107 mg

40. Corn Bread

Preparation Time: 10 minutes

Cooking Time: 20 minutes

Servings: 10

Ingredients:

- Cooking spray for greasing the baking dish
- 1 1/4 cups yellow cornmeal
- 3/4 cup all-purpose flour
- 1 tbsp. Baking soda substitute
- 1/2 cup Granulated sugar
- 2 Eggs
- 1 cup Unsweetened, unfortified rice milk –
- 2 tbsp. olive oil

Directions:

1. Heat an oven to 425F.
2. Lightly spray an 8-by-8-inch baking dish w/ cooking spray. Set aside.
3. In a medium bowl, stir together the cornmeal, flour, baking soda substitute, and sugar.
4. In a small bowl, whisk together the eggs, rice milk, and olive oil until blended.
5. Add the wet ingredients to dry ingredients and stir until well combined.
6. Pour the batter into baking dish and bake for 20 minutes or until golden and cooked through.
7. Serve warm.

Nutrition:

Calories: 198

Fat: 5g

Carbs: 34g

Phosphorus: 88mg

Potassium: 94mg

Sodium: 25mg

Protein: 4g

41. Vegetable Rolls

Preparation Time: 30 minutes

Cooking Time: 0 minutes

Servings: 8

Ingredients:

- 1/2 cup finely shredded red cabbage
- 1/2 cup grated carrot
- 1/4 cup julienne red bell pepper
- 1/4 cup julienned scallion, both green and white parts
- 1/4 cup chopped cilantro
- 1 tbsp. olive oil
- 1/4 tsp ground cumin
- 1/4 tsp freshly ground black pepper –
- English cucumber – 1, sliced very thin strips

Directions:

1. In a bowl, toss together the black pepper, cumin, olive oil, cilantro, scallion, red pepper, carrot, and cabbage. Mix well.
2. Evenly divide the vegetable filling among the cucumber strips, placing the filling close to one end of the strip.
3. Roll up the cucumber strips around the filling and secure with a wooden pick.
4. Repeat with each cucumber strip.

Nutrition:
Calories: 26

Fat: 2g

Carbs: 3g

Phosphorus: 14mg

Potassium: 95mg

Sodium: 7mg

Protein: 0g

42. Frittata with Penne

Preparation Time: 15 minutes

Cooking Time: 30 minutes

Servings: 4

Ingredients:

- 6 Egg whites
- 1/4 cup Rice milk
- 1 tbsp. chopped fresh parsley
- 1 tsp chopped fresh thyme
- 1 tsp. chopped fresh chives
- Ground black pepper
- 2 tsp olive oil
- 1/4 small sweet onion, chopped
- 1 tsp minced garlic
- 1/2 cup boiled and chopped red bell pepper
- 2 cups cooked penne

Directions:

1. Heat an oven to 350F.
2. In a bowl, whisk the egg whites, rice milk, parsley, thyme, chives, and pepper.
3. Heat the oil in a skillet.
4. Sauté the onion, garlic, red pepper for 4 minutes or until they are softened
5. Add the cooked penne to the skillet.
6. Pour the egg mixture over the pasta and shake the pan to coat the pasta.

7. Leave the skillet on the heat for 1 minute to set the bottom of the frittata and then transfer the skillet to the oven.
8. Bake, the frittata for 25 minutes or until it is set and golden brown.
9. Serve.

Nutrition:

Calories: 170

Fat: 3g

Carbs: 25g

Phosphorus: 62mg

Potassium: 144mg

Sodium: 90mg

Protein: 10g

43. Grilled Zucchini Hummus

Preparation Time: 10 minutes

Cooking Time: 10 minutes

Servings: 4

Ingredients:

- 4 zucchinis, halved
- 1/4 tsp paprika
- 1/4 cup fresh cilantro
- 1 tsp cumin
- 2 1/2 tbsp. tahini
- 2 tbsp. fresh lemon juice
- 1 tbsp. olive oil
- 2 garlic cloves, peeled
- Pepper
- Salt

Directions:

1. Season the zucchini with pepper and salt. Arrange zucchini on hot grill and cook for 10 minutes.
2. Transfer grilled zucchini along with ingredients into the food processor and process until smooth. Serve and enjoy.

Nutrition:

Calories 136

Fat 10 g

Carbs 9g

Sugar 3g

Protein 4g

Cholesterol 0mg

Phosphorus 91 mg

Potassium 159 mg

Sodium 14 mg

44. Zucchini Tots

Preparation Time: 10 minutes

Cooking Time: 20 minutes

Servings: 4

Ingredients:

- 2 eggs, lightly beaten
- 2 cups zucchini grated and squeeze out all liquid
- 1/2 cup cheddar cheese, shredded
- 2 tbsp. onion, minced
- 1/2 cup parmesan cheese, grated
- Pepper
- Salt

Directions:

1. Heat an oven to 400 F. Spry mini muffin trays with cooking spray and set aside. Add all ingredients into the bowl and mix until well combined.
2. Pour batter into the prepared muffin tray and bake for 20 minutes. Serve and enjoy.

Nutrition:

Calories 100

Fat 7g

Carbs 3g

Sugar 2g

Protein 7g

Cholesterol 95 mg

Phosphorus 157 mg

Potassium 255 mg

Sodium 389 mg

45. Stuffed Mushrooms

Preparation Time: 10 minutes

Cooking Time: 25 minutes

Servings: 4

Ingredients:

- 12 mushrooms, clean and cut stems
- 8 oz. cream cheese
- 1 tbsp. butter
- 3 bacon slices, cooked and chopped
- 2 tbsp. chives, chopped
- 1/2 tsp paprika
- Pepper
- Salt

Directions:

1. Heat an oven to 400 F.
2. Finely chop the mushroom stems.
3. Melt butter into the pan over medium heat. Add chopped mushroom stems and sauté for a minute. Remove from heat. In a bowl, mix together cream cheese, bacon, sautéed mushroom stems, chives, paprika, pepper, and salt. Stuff cream cheese mixture into each mushroom and arrange mushrooms in a baking dish. Bake in preheated oven for 20 minutes. Serve and enjoy.

Nutrition:

Calories 313

Fat 28.8g

Carbs 3.7g

Sugar 1.1g

Protein 11.4g

Cholesterol 86mg

Phosphorus 126 mg

Potassium 378 mg

Sodium 364 mg

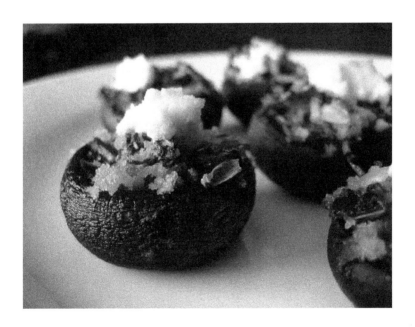

46. Tasty Herb Dip

Preparation Time: 10 minutes

Cooking Time: 5 minutes

Servings: 8

Ingredients:

- 1 cup mayonnaise
- 1 tsp dried dill
- 1 tsp dried parsley
- 1 tsp dried chives
- 1/2 cup sour cream
- 1/2 tsp onion powder
- 1/2 tsp garlic powder
- Pepper
- Salt

Directions:

1. Add all ingredients into the bowl and mix until well combined. Place in refrigerator for 20 minutes.
2. Serve and enjoy.

Nutrition:

Calories 143

Fat 12g

Carbs 8g

Sugar 2g

Protein 1g

Cholesterol 15mg

Phosphorus 30 mg

Potassium 78 mg

Sodium 245 mg

47. Rutabaga Wedges

Preparation Time: 10 minutes

Cooking Time: 20 minutes

Servings: 4

Ingredients:

- 1 lb. rutabaga, peel and cut into wedges
- 3 tbsp. olive oil
- 1/2 tsp paprika
- 1/4 tsp garlic powder
- Pepper
- Salt

Directions:

1. Heat an oven to 400 F.
2. Add rutabaga wedges into the mixing bowl. Add remaining ingredients on top and toss to coat.
3. Transfer rutabaga wedges on a baking tray and bake in preheated oven for 20 minutes.
4. Serve and enjoy.

Nutrition:

Calories 163

Fat 14g

Carbs 9g

Sugar 6g

Protein 2g

Cholesterol 0 mg

Phosphorus 67 mg

Potassium 393 mg

Sodium 15 mg

48. Tasty Broccoli Nuggets

Preparation Time: 10 minutes

Cooking Time: 30 minutes

Servings: 4

Ingredients:

- 2 cups broccoli florets
- 2 egg whites
- 1/4 cup almond flour
- 1 cup cheddar cheese, shredded
- Salt

Directions:

1. Heat an oven to 350 F.
2. Add broccoli into the boiling water and cook for 10 minutes or until softened. Drain well.
3. Spray a baking tray with cooking spray and set aside.
4. Add cooked broccoli florets into the large bowl and using potato masher mash into small pieces.
5. Add remaining ingredients and mix until well combined.
6. Make small nuggets from mixture place onto the baking tray and bake for 20 minutes.
7. Serve and enjoy.

Nutrition:

Calories 175

Fat 14g

Carbs 5g

Sugar 1g

Protein 11g

Cholesterol 30 mg

Phosphorus 17 mg

Potassium 67 mg

Sodium 34 mg

49. Onion Dip

Preparation Time: 10 minutes

Cooking Time: 4 hours 30 minutes

Servings: 12

Ingredients:

- 4 onions, sliced
- 2 tbsp. olive oil
- 2 tbsp. butter
- 1/2 cup mozzarella cheese
- 8 oz. sour cream
- Pepper
- Salt

Directions:

1. Add oil, butter, and onions into the crock pot and stir well.
2. Cover and cook on high for 4 hours.
3. Transfer onion mixture into the blender with sour cream, pepper, and salt and blend until smooth.
4. Return blended onion mixture into the crock pot.
5. Add mozzarella cheese and stir well and cook on low for 30 minutes more.
6. Stir and serve.

Nutrition:

Calories 96

Fat 8g

Carbs 4g

Protein 2g

Cholesterol 15mg

Phosphorus 47 mg

Potassium 63 mg

Sodium 66 mg

50. Beef Salad

Preparation Time: 15 minutes

Cooking Time: 35 minutes

Servings: 1

Ingredients:

- 8 cups torn romaine lettuce
- 1/2 cup each julienned cucumber, sweet yellow pepper, and red onion
- 4 teaspoon canola oil
- 1/2 cup of halved grape tomatoes
- Chili-lime vinaigrette
- 1/4 cup fresh lime juice
- 1 teaspoon of grated lime rind
- 1 tablespoon honey
- 1 tablespoon Asian chili sauce
- 2 tablespoon rice vinegar
- 1 tablespoon minced ginger root
- 1 tablespoon fresh lime juice
- 1 tablespoon cornstarch
- 1 teaspoon Asian chili sauce
- 2 cloves garlic, minced
- 1 lb. Beef Strip Loin, Top Sirloin or Flank Steak, thinly sliced

Directions:

1. Combine the chili sauce, sesame oil, garlic, lime juice, ginger root, and cornstarch in a medium bowl.

2. Add beef. Toss to coat. Let stand for 10 minutes.

3. In a large fry pan, heat 1 teaspoon canola oil.

4. Stir-fry onion, yellow pepper, cucumber, tomatoes until just wilted and hot. Transfer to the clean bowl.

5. Heat remaining canola oil in the same pan. Stir-fry beef until cooked and browned.

6. Add to wilted vegetables, tossing to combine.

7. Whisk all chili-lime vinaigrette ingredients together.

8. Put chili-lime vinaigrette in the pan. Cook until hot and slightly thickened.

9. Top romaine with veggies and beef and vinaigrette.

Nutrition:

Protein - 13g;

Phosphorus: 36mg;

Potassium: 194mg;

Sodium: 31mg;

Carbs - 6g;

Fat - 4.3g;

Calories – 116

Conclusion

Managing chronic kidney disease (CKD) requires lifestyle adjustments, but it might help to know that you're not alone. Over 31 m. Individuals in the United States are detected with malfunctions of their kidneys or are battling kidney disease. I have helped many people manage the physical symptoms associated with this disease and cope with the emotional toll that this life change can take. Without knowing what the future holds, uncertainty, fear, depression, and anxiety can be common. It may even feel like dialysis is inevitable, and you may be asking yourself if it is worth the time or effort to try and manage this stage of the disease, or if it's even possible to delay the progression. As an expert in this field, I can assure you it is not just possible, it's yours to achieve—only 1 in 50 diagnosed with CKD end up on dialysis. So together, with the right tools, we can work to delay and ultimately prevent end-stage renal disease and dialysis. Success is earned through diet modifications and lifestyle changes. Using simple, manageable strategies, I have watched firsthand as my patients empowered themselves with knowledge. They have gone on to lead full, productive, and happy lives, continuing to work, play, and enjoy spending time with their loved ones—just the way it should be!

Only 1 in 50 diagnosed with CKD end up on dialysis

Diet is a vital part of treatment for CKD, and it can help immensely in slowing the progression of the disease. Some ingredients help the kidneys function, while others make the kidneys work harder. This book has focused on crowding out the unhealthy with healthy and helpful. Also, targeting factors like salt and carbohydrate intake are important to reduce the risk of hypertension, diabetes, and other diseases that can result from kidney failure. I can't emphasize enough the importance of consulting a dietitian throughout CKD progression to optimize health. This book is a good start, as it is designed specifically for the treatment of this population.

In this time of change and uncertainty, the knowledge you gain from these pages will give you the power to take your life into your hands and make changes to benefit you in the short and long term. I hope to educate & inspire you with new, easy ways to change your health trajectory. Adopting a kidney-friendly lifestyle can be challenging at first but following these recipes will reduce the anxiety associated with selecting smart food options for your everyday life. And lest you worry that your new diet is restrictive or unsustainable, I want to assure you that these recipes are both easy and delicious, and they will give you a realistic, satisfying way to make this lifestyle change. This book will be your guide you at each step of the way. Doing so will help take the stress of meal planning out of the equation and help you focus on the truly important things in life.

Conversion Tables

Volume Equivalents (Liquid)

US STANDARD	US STANDARD (OUNCES)	METRIC (APPROXIMATE)
2 tablespoons	1 fl. oz.	30 mL
1/4 cup	2 fl. oz.	60 mL
1/2 cup	4 fl. oz.	120 mL
1 cup	8 fl. oz.	240 mL
1 1/2 cups	12 fl. oz.	355 mL
2 cups or 1 pint	16 fl. oz.	475 mL
4 cups or 1 quart	32 fl. oz.	1 L
1 gallon	128 fl. oz.	4 L

Volume Equivalents (Dry)

US STANDARD	METRIC (APPROXIMATE)
1/4 teaspoon	1 mL
1/2 teaspoon	2 mL
1 teaspoon	5 mL
1 tablespoon	15 mL
1/4 cup	59 mL
cup	79 mL
1/2 cup	118 mL
1 cup	177 mL

Oven Temperatures

FAHRENHEIT (F)	CELSIUS (C) (APPROXIMATE)
250°F	120 °C
300°F	150°C
325°F	165°C
350°F	180°C
375°F	190°C
400°F	200°C
425°F	220°C
450°F	230°C

Weight Equivalents

US STANDARD	METRIC (APPROXIMATE)
1/2 ounce	15 g
1 ounce	30 g
2 ounces	60 g
4 ounces	115 g
8 ounces	225 g
12 ounces	340 g
16 ounces or 1 pound	455 g

References

American Diabetes Association. "Age, Race, Gender & Family History." February 12, 2014. Accessed June 15, 2015. http://www.diabetes.org/are-you-at-risk/lower-your-risk/nonmodifiables.html.

American Dietetic Association. "Pocket Resource for Nutrition Assessment: 2009 Edition." 2009. Accessed June 16, 2015. http://dpg-storage.s3.amazonaws.com/dhcc/resources/PocketResources/PRNA%202009.pdf.

American Kidney Fund. "Kidney Disease Statistics." Accessed June 14, 2015. http://www.kidneyfund.org/about-us/assets/pdfs/akf-kidneydiseasestatistics-2012.pdf.

American Kidney Fund. "Race/Ethnicity and Kidney Disease." Accessed June 15, 2015. http://www.kidneyfund.org/are-you-at-risk/risk-factors/race-kidney-disease.

Centers for Disease Control and Prevention. "National Chronic Kidney Disease Fact Sheet, 2014." 2014. Accessed June 16, 2015. http://www.cdc.gov/diabetes/pubs/pdf/kidney_factsheet.pdf.

Clinical Journal of the American Society of Nephrology. "Prevalence of Chronic Kidney Disease in US Adults with Undiagnosed Diabetes or Prediabetes." January 8, 2010. Accessed June 14, 2015. http://cjasn.asnjournals.org/content/5/4/673.

DaVita HealthCare Partners. "Phosphorus and Chronic Kidney Disease." Accessed June 18, 2015. http://www.davita.com/kidney-disease/diet-and-nutrition/diet-basics/phosphorus-and-chronic-kidney-disease/e/5306.

DaVita HealthCare Partners. "Potassium and Chronic Kidney Disease." Accessed June 18, 2015. http://www.davita.com/kidney-disease/diet-and-nutrition/diet%20basics/potassium-and-chronic-kidney-disease/e/5308.

Kidney & Urology Foundation of America. "High Blood Pressure and Kidney Disease." August 2005. Accessed June 16, 2015. http://www.kidneyurology.org/Library/Kidney_Health/High_Blood_Pressure_and_Kidney_Disease.php.

Krishnamurthy, V., G. Wei, B. Baird, M. Murtaugh, M. Chonchol, K. Raphael, T. Greene, S. Beddhu. "High Dietary Fiber Intake Is Associated w/ Decreased Inflammation and All-Cause Mortality In Patients with Chronic Kidney Disease." Kidney International, 81 (3: February 2012), 300–6. Doi: 10.1038/ki.2011.355.

National Institute of Diabetes & Digestive & Kidney Diseases. "Kidney Disease of Diabetes." April 2, 2004. Accessed June 15, 2015. http://www.niddk.nih.gov/health-information/health-topics/kidney-disease/kidney-disease-of-diabetes/Pages/facts.aspx.

National Institutes of Health. "Kidney Disease: Early Detection and Treatment." NIH Medline plus 3, number 1 (winter 2008): 9–10. Accessed June 15, 2015. http://www.nlm.nih.gov/medlineplus/magazine/issues/winter08/articles/winter08pg9-10.html.

National Kidney Foundation. "About Chronic Kidney Disease." Accessed July 12, 2015. https://www.kidney.org/kidneydisease/aboutckd.

National Kidney Foundation. "Cholesterol and Chronic Kidney Disease." Accessed June 16, 2015. https://www.kidney.org/atoz/content/cholesterol.

National Kidney Foundation. "How Your Kidneys Work." Accessed June 15, 2015. https://www.kidney.org/kidneydisease/howkidneyswrk.

National Kidney Foundation. "KDOQI Clinical Practice Guidelines & Clinical Practice Recommendations for Diabetes & Chronic Kidney Disease." Accessed June 16, 2015. http://www2.kidney.org/professionals/KDOQI/guideline_diabetes/guide5.htm.

National Kidney Foundation. "Phosphorus and Your CKD Diet." Accessed June 16, 2015. https://www.kidney.org/atoz/content/phosphorus.

National Kidney Foundation. "Sodium and Your CKD Diet: How to Spice up Your Cooking." Accessed June 17, 2015. https://www.kidney.org/atoz/content/sodiumckd.

National Kidney Foundation. "Vitamins and Minerals in Kidney Disease." Accessed June 17, 2015. https://www.kidney.org/atoz/content/vitamineral.

The Renal Association. "CKD Stages." Accessed June 16, 2015. http://www.renal.org/information-resources/the-uk-eckd-guide/ckd-stages#sthash.jWT6jJfH.dpbs.

Renal Health Network. "Are Your Kidneys Okay?" Accessed June 15, 2015. http://www.renalhealthnetwork.com/index.php?page=are-your-kidneys-okay.

US Department of Agriculture. "National Agriculture Library: Macronutrients." Accessed June 16, 2015. http://fnic.nal.usda.gov/food-composition/macronutrients.

US Department of Agriculture. "National Nutrient Database for Standard Reference Release 27." Accessed June 16, 2015. http://ndb.nal.usda.gov.

US National Library of Medicine. "Medline Plus: Chronic Kidney Disease." October 2, 2013. Accessed June 16, 2015. http://www.nlm.nih.gov/medlineplus/ency/article/000471.htm.

Credits

CPSIA information can be obtained
at www.ICGtesting.com
Printed in the USA
BVHW011502160221
600148BV00024B/32